Mindfulness Journal for Mental Health

Mindfulness Journal for Mental Health

Prompts and Practices to Improve
Your Well-Being

Elizabeth Cronin, PsyD

ROCKRIDGE
PRESS

For general information on our other products and services or to obtain technical support, please contact our Customer Care Department within the United States at (866) 744-2665, or outside the United States at (510) 253-0500.

Rockridge Press publishes its books in a variety of electronic and print formats. Some content that appears in print may not be available in electronic books, and vice versa.

TRADEMARKS: Rockridge Press and the Rockridge Press logo are trademarks or registered trademarks of Callisto Media Inc. and/or its affiliates, in the United States and other countries, and may not be used without written permission. All other trademarks are the property of their respective owners. Rockridge Press is not associated with any product or vendor mentioned in this book.

Interior and Cover Designer: Linda Kocur
Art Producer: Melissa Malinowsky
Production Editor: Jax Berman
Production Manager: Martin Worthington

© Maria Galybina/Creative Market, cover; All other illustrations used under license from Paper Cards/ Creative Market. Author photo courtesy of Laura Lee Creative

Paperback ISBN: 978-1-63878-094-6
R0

This journal belongs to

Kristin

Contents

Introduction

Welcome! If you're reading this, you're probably looking for a resource to help you manage your mental health—and you are not alone. We all face challenges to our mental health, and while we can't avoid them, we can choose how we respond.

As a clinical psychologist and certified mindfulness meditation teacher, I know that practicing mindfulness can improve mental health. I've worked with individuals dealing with depression, anxiety, and other mental health issues, and I have seen them use mindfulness practices to heal and grow. In my own personal struggles with mental health, I've gained a first-person perspective on how becoming mindful can improve one's well-being. I am excited to introduce you to practices, prompts, and affirmations so you can begin to engage with mindfulness.

Mental health is important, and when it is compromised, we suffer. Numerous symptoms may develop, including trouble concentrating, problems with sleep and appetite, and relationship difficulties. You may be experiencing symptoms now—perhaps you're feeling overwhelmed, irritable, unmotivated, or discouraged.

Difficult emotions are a part of life, but when they dominate our daily lives, we experience "dis-ease," or mental illness. According to the 2021 *State of Mental Health in America* report, the number of people reporting high levels of anxiety continues to rise. Stress and anxiety are key factors in both physical and mental illness. When our mental health is compromised, we end up on autopilot, putting one foot in front of the other, just trying to survive.

But we don't have to live like this. We can learn to use mindfulness to control how we respond to stress. Over the past 20 years, a mountain of research, including work by psychologists Christopher Germer and Kristin Neff, has documented the benefits of mindfulness. Additionally, recent research has found that our brain's neuroplasticity—its ability to remain flexible and respond to change—is active not just during childhood but in all stages of life.

The guided mindfulness practices in this journal provide an excellent way to take advantage of that neuroplasticity to "re-wire" your brain. Using this journal, you can explore ways to encourage healthier thinking patterns and deepen your self-awareness. Just by reading this far, you are already one step closer to improving your mental health and well-being.

How to Use This Book

This journal uses guided mindfulness practices, prompts, and positive affirmations to support your mental health. The **prompts** pose thought-provoking questions to foster self-exploration through writing. The **practices** offer exercises and reflection space to help you become more aware of your present self. The **affirmations** provide a reminder of the bigger picture to support your work toward improved well-being. Each exercise is intended to encourage reflection and help you pause and allow yourself perspective. If you don't like the sound of a given activity, I urge you to let go of judgment and try it anyway.

Each of the three parts of this journal addresses a component of mental health. The exercises do not require prior knowledge of mindfulness, but they will challenge those who do have previous experience.

Part I dives deep into emotions. This section will help us become more aware of how examining our feelings can offer insight into ourselves and our values.

Part II examines the way our thoughts influence our decisions. This section offers mindfulness practices to support positive changes in our thinking patterns.

Part III explores how practicing mindfulness benefits our relationship with ourselves and with others. This section will help us navigate social situations with greater awareness and presence.

You'll get the most out of this journal if you work through it in order. The topics and practices at the beginning of each part set a foundation for those later on, so avoid skipping around.

Remember that while a guided mindfulness practice journal can support improvements in mental health, it is not a replacement for therapy, medication, or medical treatment. If you experience persistent difficult feelings, please contact a medical professional. We can all benefit from the support of a caring clinician.

Before you turn the page, take a moment to appreciate yourself for being open to this journey. Your willingness to take specific steps toward improving your well-being has already begun!

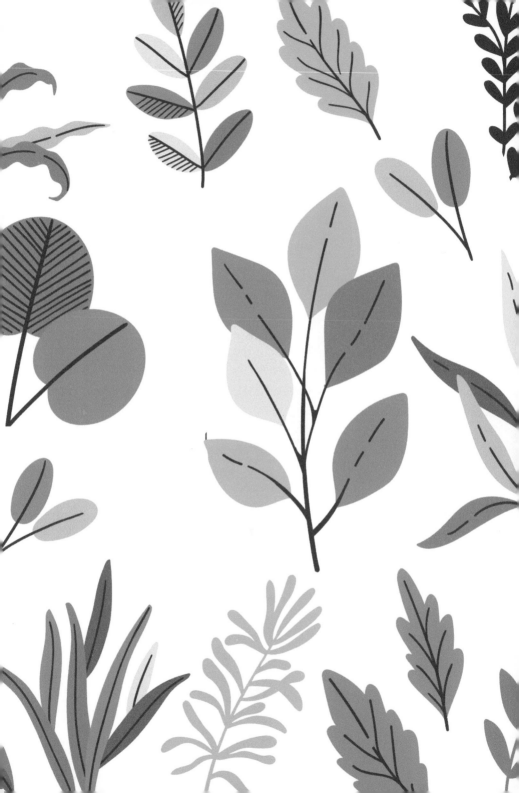

Embrace Your Emotions

IN PART I, we explore how mindfulness practices can help us understand and manage our feelings.

As human beings, it's our nature to avoid pain and pursue pleasure. We don't tolerate intense negative emotions well, and when they arise, we often try to protect ourselves by ignoring, avoiding, numbing, or denying them. As soon as we're uncomfortable, we jump into prediction, planning, and/or problem-solving mode. But in our automatic effort to dodge difficult feelings, we unintentionally skip the step of processing the emotion itself, which may cause pain and suffering down the line.

Mindfulness is helpful here in learning to slow down our automatic reactions. It allows us to notice a feeling and create space to consider our options. There are four well-established therapies that incorporate mindfulness. The most well-known are Mindfulness-Based Stress Reduction (MBSR), Dialectical Behavior Therapy (DBT), and Mindfulness-Based Cognitive Therapy (MBCT), all introduced in the late 1970s. More recently, Acceptance and Commitment Therapy (ACT) has gained popularity.

The exercises in part I are influenced by these therapies. The practices, prompts, and affirmations focus on using mindfulness exercises to recognize and reframe our emotions. Positive change is possible, so get out a pen and jump right in!

Writing down our intentions increases our chances of following through. Take time here to reflect upon your motivation for using this journal. Can you commit to trying practices, even if they seem unusual? How will you support yourself to work through to the end?

I am motivated to use this journal to exorcize childhood traumas to break down to threats, broken promises and punishments

I want to discover the way they may be used in childhood trauma as motivators

I'd like to see how that we stopped abusing children in this continue as opposed to recent generations

Abuse of students/children is never Allowable, Protection of the student is my primary concern. It hurts my heart to see bullying and hateful exclusion of staff + students.

When it comes to me and seeing someone excluded, it makes me want to sit with that person so they aren't alone.

The excluded student is a bit more complicated. Since I'm the adult, I cannot be a peer. I may be able to share stories that may relate to the conflict or issue at hand.

I want to be a better person for myself so I can enjoy others and commit to a community. I've felt so alone my whole life. Trying to be me and be myself in front of others has been hard for me. I've always been rejected from my peers for unknown reasons no one has told me about. So I feel lost when I want to know how to act. I'd like to fit in, but not in a superficial way. I'd like honest friendships again.

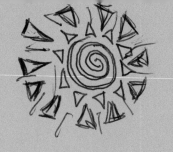

I am open
to learning new ideas,
and I look forward to a
better understanding
of myself and my
emotions.
—True

Mindfulness of Eating

Part of becoming mindful is learning to observe the intricate details of everyday life. At your next meal, pay attention to small aspects of the experience. Remove distractions and focus on your meal and only your meal. (If you're uncomfortable focusing on eating, apply the same exercise to taking a mindful shower or bath.)

Start by taking a good look at the food on your plate (or the items in your bath). What colors do you see? What textures? What do you smell? What do you taste? Do you enjoy one flavor more than another? Why?

As you eat, see if you can determine a point when you begin to feel satiated. What does it feel like? What specific bodily sensations signal to you that you've had enough?

Did you discover anything new during this experience?

When we are distracted, by definition, we can't enjoy the present moment. For instance, have you ever played your favorite song and had to hit repeat when you realized you didn't hear it the first time? What are some examples of this type of distraction experience in your life?

I feel distracted when I have too much going on in my head. I know this is part of my anxiety and that it is not rational to complete all of the tasks at once as they seem to pile on as soon as the day begins.

I can be in the present moment to enjoy simple things such as being in nature. By taking a walk or a hike, this allows me to take in the elements and the beauty around me. I don't enjoy being alone at these times. I love sharing simple moments to be present with someone I love. Jeff and I can enjoy walks together on nature hikes just to connect with each other and talk about or plans for the future with each other. Those are the times I enjoy with him most.

I need to slow down my day:

1. Prioritize my day with a planner

2. Checklists are great I love crossing items off my to do list

3. Give each item on the agenda equal time with equal attention without getting too involved in the details

4. If I cannot completely give my attention to an impatient person/item, reschedule a better time or ask for help you fool!

5. You can't do everything by yourself, Kristin. Give yourself grace.

Smile More, Stress Less

The saying "grin and bear it" suggests that smiling through difficulty helps us tolerate pain. A research group at the University of Kansas recruited participants for a study to examine how smiling affects our recovery from stress. They asked individuals to perform a task with their non-dominant hand, which raised the participants' heart rates. Those who were instructed to smile throughout the exercise had lower heart rates after recovering from the task than those who maintained a neutral expression. The act of smiling, even when instructed, triggers the release of ~~enzymes~~ hormones that reduce stress and lower the heart rate.

So the next time you notice yourself bracing for bad news or dreading making a difficult phone call, try gently smiling before and during. (A small smile works—you don't have to grin.) If it doesn't feel helpful the first time you try it, don't be discouraged. There may be some tasks that lend themselves more organically to this smiling technique. Experiment and record what works for you.

We know that smiling helps soothe our nervous system after we've experienced stress. Use this space to make a list of the things that make you smile. How can you incorporate more of these into your daily routine?

Taking Note of Emotions

Most of us spend our days going through the motions, often unaware of what we are feeling. We are used to being guided by our thoughts and disconnected from our emotions. For instance, it may take getting a headache to help us realize we are tired or hungry. We can learn a lot about ourselves by using mindful awareness to check in with how we feel in different settings, at certain times of day, or with specific people.

Choose a day when you can schedule a one-minute pause every two to four hours. Set an alarm to go off at your chosen intervals, and keep paper handy to record notes. When you hear the alarm, stop what you are doing and ask yourself these questions:

- How am I feeling right now?

- Where am I?

- What am I doing?

- Who am I with?

- Why am I doing what I'm doing?

Record your answers and any other relevant details.

Review the emotions in the record of your day of mindful awareness. What patterns do you notice? Did your emotions change based on the who, what, where, and/or why of the situation?

Emotions as Messages

Embracing our emotions is easier when we view them as messages toward rather than reflections of ourselves. Just as a message contains information for its recipient, emotions communicate information about our current situation. Mindfulness-based therapies help draw connections between our emotions and the "messages" they are communicating. For example, fear alerts us that we perceive danger. Confusion indicates a need for direction or guidance. Anger signals an unmet need or a violation of boundaries. Sadness communicates that something we value is absent or lost. Joy lets us know we are engaged in something pleasurable.

Emotions provide clues to who we are and what we desire. When we ignore unpleasant feelings, we miss an opportunity to identify and fulfill an unmet need. When you experience an emotion, pause, stay with it, and allow yourself to wonder what information it is communicating. Reflect on your experience here.

_____

_____

_____

_____

_____

_____

_____

_____

_____

_____

_____

_____

_____

_____

_____

_____

_____

_____

_____

_____

_____

_____

_____

_____

My emotions bring
me information.
I make space to
explore their messages
before reacting.

Just as hunger reminds us to eat and fatigue indicates a need for sleep, our emotions provide information. What emotions do you experience on a regular basis? What messages might they be trying to convey?

What We Resist Will Persist

This practice asks you to add another layer to your mindfulness by noticing when you're resisting or avoiding an emotion. Trying to suppress our emotions creates pressure, like a secret we can't share. We hold tension in our bodies when we try to stifle an intense feeling.

But pushing away problematic feelings isn't healthy (or helpful) long-term. The effort of resisting our emotions triggers a stress response, and our body releases chemicals intended to help us fight or escape. If this happens regularly, it can contribute to physical and/or mental illnesses, including high blood pressure and heart disease.

As you continue to notice the ebb and flow of emotions throughout your day, pay attention to any instances when you recognize a reluctance to experience your feeling. Note physical signs of stress, such as increased heart rate, rapid breathing, sweating, and/or shakiness.

Check-In

As you make your way through this journal, you'll encounter more practice exercises that connect you with "easy" emotions and difficult ones. At this point in your journey, which emotions do you find most difficult to tolerate?

Increase Pleasurable Activities

Being mindful requires us to understand that there are some things we can't control. Dealing with adversity is a part of life—and hardship from time to time is inevitable, no matter how hard we work or how thoroughly we plan.

While we can't prevent hardship altogether, we can work to balance it with pleasurable activities that *are* within our control, such as:

- Playing music
- Noticing pleasant fragrances (like flowers or candles)
- Going outside for fresh air
- Hugging someone we care for
- Lighting a candle
- Preparing a favorite beverage
- Reading
- Enjoying a warm bath/shower

Reflect on how you can bring more simple, pleasurable experiences into your life. What are some things that you already have access to that can bring you more pleasure if you pause to allow it in?

Knowing that incorporating pleasure into our daily lives improves our well-being, what things can you do every day to add joy to your routine?

_____

_____

_____

_____

_____

_____

_____

_____

_____

_____

_____

_____

_____

_____

_____

I can manage
my emotions
by incorporating
activities I enjoy,
and I remember
to give thanks for all
that I already have.

Change Your Mood with Gratitude

Our moods are influenced by where we direct our attention. When we notice that someone has something we want, jealousy arises. If we look for flaws, we may feel disappointed or embarrassed. In our attempt to stay safe, we're on constant alert for trouble, thinking it gives us an advantage. Instead, it sets us up for suffering: In fixating on problems to solve, we overlook what's positive.

Shifting our attention toward what we already have is a powerful way to improve mood and shift perspective. A gratitude practice is a great mindfulness exercise to add to your daily routine.

Choose a time during your daily routine to make a mental gratitude list of all that you appreciate. You can count your relationships, character traits, experiences, talents, skills, and even possessions.

In our busy lives, we take all kinds of things for granted—our health, friends, neighbors, access to transportation, television, technology, and so on. What things in your life are you grateful for? What would you miss if it were gone tomorrow?

Emotions—Energy in Motion

The word "emotion" comes from the Latin *emotere*, which means "energy in motion." Our senses absorb information about a given situation, prompting our emotional response. These pleasant or painful signals move through our bodies as energy seeking release.

When we feel frightened, adrenaline provides extra energy needed to fight or escape a situation. When we feel sad, our bodies create tears. If we allow this process, our emotions are like waves, ebbing and flowing according to our situation.

But if our emotions are suppressed, or otherwise not appropriately released, the suppressed energy builds up and can resurface later as an outburst. Rather than trying to ignore or hide our emotions, we can learn to release the energy in a healthy way. Yoga, exercise, talking, acupuncture, and meditation are all popular outlets.

Take 5 to 10 minutes to reflect on how you release your emotions. What works best for intense feelings?

Reflect on a time when you felt strong emotions. What and where was the first sensation? What words describe the energy moving through your body? (Pulsing, tingling, throbbing, clenching?) How long did the sensations last?

You Are Not Your Emotions

A mindfulness-informed understanding of emotions recognizes that we are not our feelings. But this understanding is not reflected in the way we tend to express emotions. Here's an example: When we notice that our face is getting hot, our heart is beating fast, and our fists are clenched, we recognize anger. It's common to then say, "I am angry." Here, we use language that suggests that we are defined by our emotion. Taken even further, we might define ourselves as "an angry person."

Given that our emotions change all the time, defining ourselves according to any feeling can compromise our self-esteem and over-simplify our situation. Defining ourselves in a negative way doesn't feel great, so take a moment to ask: "*How do I feel when I say I am angry, sad, lonely, and so on?*"

A healthier way of expressing our feelings is, "*At this moment, I am feeling anger,*" or, "*Right now, I am feeling lonely.*" This small shift in language can make a big difference in your self-perception. See how it feels to allow some space between you and your emotions.

Pick three or four emotions that you struggle with and write them down. Now, practice writing out how you can express the feeling in a way that is separate from you. Do you notice a difference?

Manage Your Mood with Yoga

One healthy way to release the energy of our emotions is with movement of the breath and body through yoga. Taking time to stretch your body and breathe deeply helps soothe the nervous system, releasing negative energy and providing a reset for the body and mind.

Try this simple yoga practice almost anywhere. Lie on your back or sit down with both arms extended on either side of your body. Get in a comfortable position, using cushions or a blanket if necessary. Keep your palms facing up. With your arms outstretched, take a full, deep breath in through your nose. Hold it for a few seconds; then exhale slowly through your mouth.

Repeat, and as you breathe in, say to yourself, "*I am.*" As you exhale, continue, saying, "*Calm and centered.*" Continue repeating this pattern for five minutes.

Get in a comfortable position, either lying or sitting. Recall an unpleasant experience from your past, allowing the details to return to your mind. Notice any tension in your body. Then, try the yoga exercise described on the previous page. How do you feel afterward? Has anything changed?

When my emotions feel difficult or intense, I choose actions or activities that soothe and calm my nervous system.

Identify Your Emotional Triggers

Most of us have certain situations or stimuli that act as emotional "triggers." Emotional triggers create sudden and intense emotions that are larger and more painful than would seem expected or necessary given the situation. Our reaction is out of proportion to the cause of our upset.

These triggers result from past painful experiences that evoked a sense of helplessness and fear. Often, triggers have their roots in our early years since, as children, we rely on others to keep us safe and manage our emotions. Regardless of age, though, when we don't get the help we need, we feel overwhelmed and helpless. We retain this painful experience as an unconscious memory, like a wound that never properly healed. When someone bumps into that old wound, it breaks open, flooding us with old unprocessed emotions.

Which situations or experiences elicit stronger-than-expected reactions in you? Can you think of anything in your past that could clue you in to the original wound? It can be helpful to ask people you trust who knew you as a child if they remember any of your difficult experiences.

Can you remember what you struggled with as a child? Did you have a hard time in school or making friends? Did your family face any hardships? Did you or a loved one have health challenges? What were your relationships like? Write down anything you remember.

Testing Reality

Identifying emotional triggers is helpful because once we rule out immediate danger, we can move on to reality testing. When you experience a strong reaction, feel the energy or tension building within your body. Recognize the emotion, name it, and consider and test the reality of the message it is sending.

Let's say you're feeling jealous, and your jealousy is sending the message that you want what someone else has. Is that message accurate? Do you really want the item, or are you caught in the habit of thinking you always need what others have?

While our emotions do send messages, our feelings are not facts. Many heated emotions cool down when we allow ourselves the space to test reality and see our circumstances in perspective.

Triggers can be tricky because once an old wound is bumped, the emotions that resurface have the same intensity as our original experience. When this happens, remember that in the present moment, you are not helpless as you once were—you have control over your reaction.

Can you think of a time when you were startled or triggered, only to discover it was a "false alarm"? What was the experience like for you? How might it help in the future to be able to pause and do a reality test?

Acting Opposite

When in a state of emotional distress, resistance is a natural automatic reaction. Our bodies tense up as a voice inside us shouts, "*NO!*" If a friend isn't listening to us, we often lash out. If a coworker doesn't deliver on a promise, we might mutter mean things under our breath. If a loved one disappoints us, we imagine ending the relationship.

Acting opposite is a strategy from Dialectical Behavior Therapy (DBT) that guides us in changing how we react. It instructs us to take the action that contradicts our initial, automatic reaction—the way we're tempted to react in the heat of the moment. It takes practice, but acting opposite gives us an opportunity to practice changing our response during stressful situations.

As you move through your week, look for opportunities to practice acting opposite. For example, you might choose to pick up your loved one's coat for them instead of yelling at them for dropping it on the floor. Start with small moments that have lower stakes, and over time, work to expand this approach to the more difficult areas of life.

What automatic reactions do you tend to have in uncomfortable situations? If you were to act opposite, what might you do? How do you think you would feel?

Grounding Activities

Grounding activities are another important concept of DBT that can help us process intense emotions. Even as we practice mindfulness, we as humans remain vulnerable to overwhelming feelings. In fact, embracing our emotions can be healthy as long as we don't let them consume us.

Intense feelings and their accompanying physiological distress cloud our thinking, reducing our ability to test reality (see page 46). That's why grounding activities can be helpful: They require our full mental and physical attention, giving us a break to cool off from a flurry of thoughts and feelings.

Any activity can be used for grounding if it engages your full attention. Focusing on one simple task or project keeps our minds from wandering into speculative "what-ifs" and impulsive reactions. Assuming that there is no imminent danger, staying in the present allows our nervous system to reset.

The next page has a list of popular grounding techniques. Circle the ones that you might use the next time you feel flooded by difficult, intense emotions, and feel free to add your own. Come back to this list as needed!

Gardening

Working on puzzles

Listening to music

Cooking

Cleaning

Calling someone

Taking a walk

Dancing

Putting on lotion

Looking out the window

Getting into nature

Hugging someone

Wrapping yourself up
in a blanket

Jumping up and down

Stretching

Doing yoga

Playing an instrument

Doing breathing exercises

Painting, coloring, or doing
another creative activity

Playing with something or
someone

Helping someone

Journaling

Singing

Bathing

Sipping a beverage

Napping

Decorating

Playing a game

Baking

Planning an outing

Organizing items

Watching a movie

Reading or listening
to a book

Check-In

Before you move on to part II, reflect on any new insights that have emerged as you've worked through part I. In what ways are you more connected with and aware of your emotions? What specific practices have helped you manage your feelings?

Cultivate Your New Mindset

IN PART II, we will examine psychological well-being, drawing connections between our thoughts and their influence on our emotions.

Psychological well-being indicates a sense of agency over one's life. Maintaining our well-being allows us to feel confident and satisfied with our decisions and actions. Because our thoughts drive our actions, it is important to look closely at our thinking mind. In this section, we'll explore how well-established negative automatic thought patterns can unconsciously impede our efforts to respond to challenges the way we want to.

Mindfulness supports our mental health by tuning us in to our brain's activity, including the unconscious assumptions and judgments we make constantly. Our thoughts function as a lens through which we interpret our lives and make decisions, so gaining control over our thoughts can open us up to make positive changes.

The practices and prompts in this section will train you to be more aware of when your mind wanders and where your thoughts go. As you make your way through the exercises, you'll learn how to slow down, take control of unwanted reactions, and live your life in the present.

We spend much of our time on autopilot, especially when we're busy. What does being on autopilot look like for you? How would you like to be more present? How might your life change?

By quieting
my mind and
becoming mindfully
aware of my thinking,
I open myself up
to positive personal
growth and
greater well-being.

Listening Meditation

When we are fully present, we're aware of the focus of our attention. We know what we are listening to and what we're tuning out. We know if our actions are being influenced by automatic negative thoughts or productive, supportive thoughts. Listening meditation can sharpen our ability to be present.

You can do this practice anywhere, sitting or standing. It should take 10 to 15 minutes. Find a comfortable space and begin breathing normally. Close your eyes or lower your gaze and focus on one spot.

Begin to pay attention to the sounds surrounding you. What can you hear? Do you hear people, pets, or traffic? Notice as many details and levels as possible. You'll likely find that you've gotten "in your head" thinking about something unrelated to the exercise. If this happens, gently return your attention to the sounds of your environment.

Our minds wander constantly, and it's easy for us to lose touch with our environment. Can you think of a time when you felt grounded in your surroundings? Where were you, who were you with, and what were you doing? How did you feel, and what can you learn from that experience?

Watching the Flickering Flame

The goal of this practice is to observe the spontaneous and random nature of your thoughts. In the spirit of loving kindness, you'll suspend your judgment and become curious, noticing and allowing whatever comes up.

Light a candle and place it where you can watch the flame flicker. Set a timer for 5 to 10 minutes and settle into a comfortable position, noticing any areas of tension within your body and allowing them to soften. Bring your attention to your breath as the air flows in and out.

As you gaze at the flame, allow your mind to wander in whatever direction it wants, opening a "stream of consciousness." Recognize the thoughts, images, and ideas that surface, but don't become attached to them—remain open to allow other thoughts to pass through. Be curious about whatever shows up, allowing your thoughts to flicker in and out of your mind. Reflect on your experience here.

Our minds are brimming with thoughts. Do any of your thoughts come up more frequently than others? Do you notice yourself evaluating, assessing, problem-solving, planning the future, or replaying the past?

Focus on Color

Our vision, like all our senses, provides information about our surroundings, and we can use the colors around us to practice mindfulness. Exercising visual attention helps us see things more clearly. With intention, we can shift how and what we see.

This practice can be done anywhere in under 10 minutes. Choose one color and look around you for instances of that color. When you find one, focus your attention on it, noticing the details. What item do you see? What is its function, shape, size, and placement? Next, move your attention to another object of the same color.

Eventually, your mind will wander, which is natural. Whenever this happens, gently return your attention to the exercise, appreciating your ability to shift your focus. This is how we become more mindful!

Different colors affect us depending on how they have shaded our experiences. What colors do you prefer, and why? How do colors brighten your life? How could you use them to bring you more pleasure?

Using Breath as an Anchor

Sitting or lying comfortably, take three deep breaths as you settle. Close your eyes or lower your gaze. Breathe naturally and stay focused on your breath, noticing the air as it enters and leaves your body. If paying attention to your breath feels uncomfortable, try focusing on the feeling of your back meeting your chair or your feet meeting the floor.

Inevitably, your mind will wander, and that's okay—just notice when it happens and return your attention to your breath. When your mind wanders again, return to breathing without judgment.

The many thoughts in our busy minds are like strong waves that rock a boat in a stormy sea. Our breath is the anchor that keeps our ship in place despite rough waters.

Reflect on your experience. How can you use breathing to keep calm amid distracting thoughts and situations?

Staying in the present
keeps me from
slipping into
autopilot, allowing me
to see things
more clearly and
to feel calm within.

Check-In

What are you learning about yourself and your thinking habits? Do you feel more capable of self-compassion as you try these new practices and challenge your problematic beliefs?

Clarify Your Values

Awareness of our thoughts and feelings gives us insight into our values. Our values, in turn, guide our decisions, helping us shape the lives we want to live. Making a list of your values can help clarify your personal preferences and strengths. Use the following questions to begin defining your values:

- Whom do you admire? What specific qualities do they exhibit?

- What positive traits have others noticed in you?

- When do you feel most proud?

- When do you feel most alive?

- What inspires you?

The answers to these questions shed light on your innate talents and unique traits. Set aside some uninterrupted time to think about these questions. You might try spending 10 minutes in quiet meditation before reflecting.

For a more in-depth exploration of your character strengths, find the link to the online Values in Action Character Strengths assessment in the Resources section (see page 157).

We all have personality traits that steer us toward and away from certain things. How have your character strengths influenced your life so far? What traits would you like to strengthen as you continue to grow?

Managing Self-Talk

The things we repeatedly tell ourselves eventually feel like the truth. While we can't change what others think or say, we can control what we think and say to ourselves, being mindful of the negative automatic chatter in our head.

Notice the automatic thoughts that pop up when you make a mistake. Dropping your keys, do you think, "*You're so stupid,*" or, "*You always do this*"? Rather than putting ourselves down for mistakes, we must address ourselves kindly, as we would a friend.

At the start of your day, commit to noticing the automatic negative commentary running in the back of your mind. Whenever you notice you're being hard on yourself, gently remind yourself that it's okay to be human. Do you notice any differences?

Think of the unhelpful negative comments you direct at yourself and write down their opposites. For example, if you say to yourself that you'll never be successful, you might write, "*I deserve to be happy and successful.*" Record your rewritten comments here. How might you feel if you spoke to yourself more compassionately?

When I speak
to myself, I am
speaking to a friend
who deserves love,
self-compassion,
and support.

Mindful Seeing

Now that you realize how frequently our minds jump from thought to thought, let's practice the skill of observing things as they are. As we take in our surroundings, our brains quickly scan for previous stimuli to inform our current scenario. We don't just see objects; we recall the thoughts and feelings associated with those objects.

Practicing seeing with a fresh perspective sheds light on the shadows of the past. As we continue to turn to this mindful seeing, we also strengthen our understanding of how our past affects the present.

Find a place with a view where you can sit comfortably for 15 minutes. Settle down and allow yourself to take in the scenery. Notice your surroundings: people, plants, cars. As soon as you begin having thoughts about your surroundings, return to pure observation without assessing anything. What are you able to see more clearly? What new observations about the scene emerge?

Being mindful leads to a greater capacity for loving kindness, the thoughtful and caring consideration of all beings (see page 111). As you practice observation without judgment, consider observing yourself with more compassion.

Write a description of yourself that celebrates the wonderful qualities that make you who you are. Don't hold back!

Beginner's Mind

Jon Kabat-Zinn, creator of the Mindfulness-Based Stress Reduction (MBSR) program, encourages us to embrace a "beginner's mind." He describes the beginner's mind as a childlike state of "not knowing" that fosters curiosity and learning.

When we are flooded with automatic negative thoughts (see page 76), we tell ourselves we "should have known" or could have prevented a given situation. In these moments, we can use a beginner's mind to let go of frustration.

Look out for a moment in your daily life when you feel pressured to "know" or be right. Notice the thoughts that come to your mind and their effect on your body. Remain present and ask yourself these questions:

Are you sure that there is one best approach or decision? Why do you need to be right or to prevent problems or uncertainty? Can you be curious about the circumstances that led to this situation?

We don't like uncertainty, and we are comforted by knowledge and information. But believing that we know everything can shut out new insights and inspiration. When is it hard for you to be uncertain or wrong? Why?

Just One Thing

At the start of your day, take a moment to commit to doing just one thing at a time. As you move from one activity to the next, remind yourself of your pledge to stay focused on one thing at a time.

If you are having lunch, then only eat lunch—avoid reading emails and scrolling on social media.

If you have a conversation, notice whether you are listening or talking, and do just one of those things at a time. If you are listening, only listen: Avoid planning your response ahead of time. If you are talking, just talk: Avoid mentally speculating on the next response.

This sounds easier than it is, but try it for a day and record some notes here.

We try to do so much every day that we often miss out on enjoying small pleasures. What small pleasures might enhance your life if you paid them more attention?

Moving Meditation

Moving or walking meditation is another way to practice mindfulness, slowing yourself down enough to notice what it's like to be in motion.

For this exercise, find a peaceful location where you can walk or move in a way that's comfortable to you without bumping into objects or people (5 to 15 feet should be enough space). Keep your eyes open and breathe naturally. As you begin to move, keep your pace slow and your movements deliberate.

Try to notice the small details that are easy to ignore. As your body moves in one direction, feel its contact with the air. What is it like when your muscles engage to propel your body forward? What sounds do you hear as you shift your weight? As you know well by now, your mind will wander, but when you notice it, return your attention to your body's movement.

As you work through these practices, have you noticed changes in your awareness of your body, thoughts, and emotions in any given situation? Write whatever comes to mind.

When I make space
for more than my
first thoughts, I see
greater possibilities,
experience more
pleasure,
and reconnect
with the present.

An Open Mind

The beginner's mind (see page 84) sees all possibilities. It doesn't limit itself to one "best" idea. The beginner's mind is an open mind—a mind willing to leave the comfort zone.

Choose an event, activity, or location that you normally avoid. Consider grocery shopping, driving kids to an activity, or visiting a museum with a friend. Pick an invitation or opportunity that you may have declined in the past. When the offer comes around this time, agree to go along. Record your notes on the following questions:

What is it like for you to participate in something you wouldn't ordinarily choose? Even if you are unhappy or uncomfortable, can you notice what you don't like? With more mindful attention, can you modify the experience to make it easier for you to continue to engage going forward?

We pursue the familiar because it's comfortable. But willingness to give something new a try—or try something again—can support our personal growth. What are two or three things that you are willing to be open to doing?

Cues for Mindful Moments

Research on habit formation indicates that cues can serve as helpful reminders to do our desired behavior. We can use this technique to remember to be mindful. When choosing a mindfulness cue, you have plenty of options in any regular day: Consider using washing your hands, answering a message, eating a meal or snack, or getting in and out of a vehicle. Anything you do multiple times a day will work.

Once you've chosen a cue, commit to using it as a reminder to pause for a moment of mindfulness. You can spend the moment in any way that feels calming to you. You might take two or three deep breaths, do some stretching, or recite some positive affirmations or a favorite poem. What cue did you choose? How did you use your mindful moment?

Check-In

Which of the practices has helped you develop or deepen your understanding of a) what it means to be present and b) how mindfulness can help you manage your mental health? What exercises can you make a part of your daily practice?

Judging Others

Mindfulness helps our perception of ourselves and our relationships with others (more on this in part III). Just as staying aware of our negative self-talk supports self-compassion (see page 76), noticing when we are judging others allows us to create more authentic connections.

We label others as bad, deficient, or harmful after we've felt hurt by their behavior. We do this to protect ourselves—but when no true threat is present, we cause ourselves unnecessary stress. While our feelings are real, our fear may, or may not, be warranted. Devoting energy to negatively labeling others leaves us anxious about unpleasant encounters, especially when it comes to those we see regularly. Here, we'll practice letting go of our judgments of others.

For this practice, go somewhere where you can observe others. As you observe, notice where your thoughts go. When you notice yourself making a judgment of someone (such as selfish, angry, foolish, etc.), pause and consider that you don't have all the information. Wonder if there is an explanation for their appearance or behavior.

Sometimes we label others because they, or their behavior, remind us of someone we already know. Can you think of times when you have made assumptions about others based on your prior experiences?

Accepting Reality

On the first page of his classic book *The Road Less Traveled*, M. Scott Peck writes that life is difficult, but that we transcend this reality by knowing and accepting this truth. The challenge comes from our aversion to pain—when we feel upset, we assume something is wrong.

Here's an example: Relationships are imperfect; they bring us joy and pain. When we accept that even the best relationships have difficult moments, we experience less distress. When we reject this truth, those difficult moments cause more pain. If we falsely believe that "good" relationships should never be difficult, we see conflict as a sign of disaster. This deepens our discomfort, leading to panic and escalation.

For this exercise, recall a situation that caused you great pain. Spend 15 minutes reflecting on the underlying expectations you had for that situation. Is there anything you could have accepted that might have helped you manage your experience of the situation and your response?

Resisting painful emotions and thoughts is part of being human—but so, too, is our greater cognitive ability to recognize our own resistance to that pain. Reflect upon and write about the things you can control in a painful situation versus what you cannot.

I am human and
mistakes are part
of life. I am worthy,
even when I am
imperfect.

Discover Improved Relationships

IN PART III, we'll explore the ways that mindfulness benefits our mental health by working on our relationship with ourselves and with others.

Understanding and managing our emotions and thoughts allows us to improve social connections, especially when we feel discomfort. The ability to stay calm despite feeling upset is a powerful form of freedom. Instead of immediately reacting to a fleeting feeling or (mis)perception, we can learn to pause, clarify the situation, and consider alternative possibilities.

Learning to challenge automatic responses can be uncomfortable, but we get better with time and practice. Staying mindful of feelings and thoughts allows us to see situations clearly before acting—a powerful way to reduce stress and deepen relationships.

Part III includes practices and prompts to support your social well-being. The exercises provide different ways to strengthen your connection with yourself and with others. These strategies can be used in personal and professional relationships, with friends and family, or with colleagues at work or school.

You will learn how mindfulness improves self-awareness, self-compassion, and your capacity to extend loving kindness to others.

Our quality of life improves when we feel connected to others. Use this space to reflect on what you believe makes a relationship healthy and connected (or unhealthy and disconnected).

I cherish my connections with others. I embrace opportunities to treat myself and others with compassion.

Loving-Kindness Meditation

Because our thoughts affect our feelings and behaviors, being critical and unfair hurts ourselves as well as others. Negativity toward oneself and others takes a toll on our relationships and well-being. The loving-kindness meditation is an antidote. We start with ourselves and work toward extending love to all beings.

Settle into a comfortable position for meditation. As you inhale and exhale, mentally recite the phrases:

May I be happy.
May I be healthy.
May I be safe.
May I live with ease.

Even if it feels mechanical, be as genuine as possible, repeating until it feels more organic. After a while, begin directing these well-wishes to someone you care about:

May you be happy.
May you be healthy.
May you be safe.
May you live with ease.

Next, direct the meditation to acquaintances, followed by strangers, and even those who may have harmed you. End the practice by sending well-wishes to all beings.

Think of someone who has supported you during difficult times. What kinds of things did they do or say that you found helpful? Describe how it felt for you.

Reflective Listening

We listen to gain insight, direction, and understanding. How we take in information affects our interactions and relationships. When we behave mindfully, we make a deliberate effort to hear not only the words someone says but the message they convey.

Without practice, it's difficult to be fully present in a conversation. Perhaps we're thinking about being somewhere else, things we need to do, or even what we want to say when it's our turn to talk. But understanding another person requires our full attention. Reflective listening can help by signaling to the other person that you are focused on them. Below are some ways to practice reflective listening:

- Maintaining eye contact

- Using non-verbal cues, like nodding

- Making short, encouraging comments, like "I see"

- Asking questions to deepen the conversation

- Summarizing what's been said

- Exhibiting affect appropriate to the content

Try this technique in your next conversation. Do you notice a difference?

Think back to an interaction when you felt unsure whether you were truly being heard. How would you describe the experience? What thoughts and emotions do you associate with this experience?

Asking for Help

Asking for help can be scary. It requires setting our egos aside and letting go of the idea that we can figure out everything on our own. Doing so may feel risky—we might worry that others will think we're weak, foolish, or lacking in experience. We might feel anxious that our request will burden someone else. We might fear that our request for help will be rejected.

Despite the imagined dangers, it's important to ask for help. We can save ourselves time and effort, expand our knowledge and resources, and spare ourselves the frustration and anxiety of failure or uncertainty. It may feel uncomfortable, but there are times when the most productive thing we can do is recognize that we would benefit from outside support.

Think of a task that feels challenging. Can you think of someone whom you could turn to for support, whether for a skill or an alternative perspective? Consider how it would feel to seek help.

Are there areas of your life in which you could use more support? What thoughts and feelings keep you from asking for help from others? How would it feel if you received help in a caring manner?

Cultivate Curiosity

When someone treats us poorly, we tend to resist and resent them. Cultivating curiosity is a way to increase our capacity for empathy. Asking questions brings understanding and reduces conflict. Instead of jumping to conclusions, we can pause, take a step back, and see the bigger picture.

In cultivating curiosity, we examine a range of possible reasons for this person's behavior and consider whether we misperceived any aspect of the interaction. We might even consider whether we unknowingly contributed in some way to the hurtful situation—after all, everyone makes mistakes. The reflection process also clarifies when resisting the harmful behavior of another is warranted.

Being mindful allows us to be aware and engaged, even when our initial reaction is discomfort. Use this technique the next time you feel mistreated or hurt, and come back and record your experience here.

I determine what
really matters to me
by choosing where I
place my attention.
I decide whom, when,
and how I can help
and whom I turn to
for support.

As children, we are innately curious. Can you remember the intrinsic awe of seeing or experiencing something for the first time? What do you think about bringing this kind of wonder into your present life?

How Can I Help You?

Helping others improves our own integrity and self-esteem. When we care for others, we like the person we are. Our innate desire to share love and be appreciated supports connection and community. In other words, helping others can help ourselves.

In everyday life, we can decide to experiment with what it's like to focus on helping someone. Choose someone you will see more than once during the day. At the start of the day, you can let them know you are doing an experiment that involves helping others. Ask them what you can specifically do for them.

Pay attention to how you feel as you engage in acts of thoughtfulness and generosity. Notice any energy in your body. You might experience shifts depending on specific tasks or the time of day. Take note of these to understand the ways you most enjoy helping others.

Check-In

Giving love, listening carefully, asking for help, and being there for others all require a level of energy that we can generate by taking care of ourselves. Which of your daily habits nourish you and replenish your energy? Can you add any?

Validating Others

This practice of validating others in conversation is a companion to reflective listening (see page 114). We express ourselves in order to be understood, so after listening to someone's communication, it's helpful to validate them. This can be challenging if we don't agree with what's said. Thinking the other is mistaken or being unfair, we might argue or correct them. But when we skip the validation step, others feel judged. By pausing to verify what's been said, we create some space to explore rather than argue.

Imagine someone says, "*Kelly is mean.*" You might not want to repeat or agree with those words. Instead, say, "*It sounds like you think Kelly is mean.*" This way, you acknowledge what was said without indicating agreement. This way of validating another sets the foundation for a healthy discussion where both parties feel heard. After validating, we can use the "cultivate curiosity" practice (see page 120) to avoid further upset.

As you go through your day, notice moments when your thoughts conflict with someone else's opinion. Instead of reactively disagreeing or staying silent, see if you can validate what's said. Notice how the conversation proceeds.

Recall a time when you tried to explain something or express your deep feelings to someone who misunderstood, minimized, or dismissed what you said. What did that feel like for you? Why is the experience upsetting? What would have helped?

I look for opportunities
to be creative,
playful, and happy.
I strive to share my joy
with all those
I encounter.

Catch Someone Doing Good

The things we pay attention to grow. Think of houseplants. When we provide them with water and sunlight, the plants flourish. People function similarly. When we notice and comment on positive choices, we reinforce and strengthen those behaviors in ourselves and others.

All too often, we focus on what's wrong or what we don't like. Those close to us notice what we notice and use this information when seeking our attention. If the easiest way to be recognized is to create a mess, that's what many will do.

But catching someone doing something "good" clarifies what we *like* to experience and promotes healthy results. It's like placing a succulent in sunshine.

Pick a person whom you may not always appreciate. In your next interaction with them, see if you can find something positive in the encounter.

When was the last time you received positive feedback on something you did? Do you remember how it felt? How do you think your relationships might change if you were to give more praise and encouragement to others?

Forgiveness

All humans make mistakes, but holding on to anger doesn't resolve anything. Forgiveness doesn't mean approving of, forgetting, or passively accepting hurt. Rather, we find peace when we stop ruminating on injustices. When we are hurt, we might take actions to protect ourselves, but accepting what happened frees up our energy and allows us to move forward.

Practicing forgiveness is somewhat like the loving-kindness meditation (see page 111). This meditation involves reciting a series of phrases silently. Pause in between statements. If you feel upset at any point, acknowledge the feeling and return to the phrases. Remember that you aren't trying to resolve problems, but rather you're creating space for forgiveness.

I am human and make mistakes. I forgive myself.
I am imperfect, and I seek forgiveness from
those I have harmed.
Everyone makes mistakes, and I have been harmed.
I offer forgiveness to those who have hurt me.

While it may feel robotic or superficial at first, this practice becomes more effective with time.

Do you find it harder to forgive yourself or others? What makes forgiveness hard for you? Can you imagine finding a way to respond to your concerns with care and kindness, helping yourself let go of past pain?

Self-Compassion Break

Self-compassion and its associated benefits are an area of interest within psychology. Dr. Kristin Neff, a leading researcher in the field, created the Self-Compassion Break, a three-step exercise to use during moments of suffering.

You can try this when you become upset, or you can use it to re-process a difficult past situation. If you're using a memory for this practice, allow yourself to feel the discomfort in your body before you begin.

Now, say to yourself:

> **I recognize and accept this moment of pain.**
> **I know I am not alone.**
> **Suffering is part of life.**

After acknowledging the above, place your hands over your heart. If this position is uncomfortable for you, choose another form of touch that feels soothing—you might try giving yourself a hug or resting your hands on your legs. Hold this pose and receive compassion from yourself.

Close the practice by asking yourself if there's anything else you need to feel better.

When you are hurting and feeling distraught, what are some ways that you can take care of yourself? Name a few things you find soothing.

Choosing Kindness

Being kind is a natural trait, but as we grow older in a competitive, often cutthroat world, kindness can be overshadowed by a tendency to hold back generosity and vulnerability. When trying to prove ourselves or get ahead in life, we forget that the kindness we offer others can be transformative.

Kindness can benefit others while boosting our well-being. In his book *Why Kindness Is Good for You*, Dr. David Hamilton writes that kindness reduces anxiety and depression, allowing us to be less distracted and more present. It also supports our connections with others, strengthening our bonds. Here are a few approaches to bring kindness back into your life—but think of some of your own, too!

- Greet those you encounter with a smile.

- Help someone who is struggling in some way.

- Let someone go ahead of you in line.

- Talk to everyone the way you would talk to a friend—yourself included.

What is the greatest act of kindness that you've ever witnessed or heard about? What were the circumstances? How has being aware of this shaped your beliefs about life?

Where I place
my attention and what
I notice is up to me.
I choose to see the
beauty in myself,
in others, and in life
all around me.

Seeking Support from Someone

Just as we all make mistakes, we all struggle with difficult situations. It may seem easier to keep these to ourselves and resolve them silently, but doing so can create stress and compromise our mental health.

By imagining that others might think less of us, we forget that turning toward another can strengthen our interpersonal connections. Reaching out to a trusted person is a healthy way to share thoughts, process feelings, and explore options.

For this practice, identify an issue that's challenged you in some way. It doesn't have to be huge, but it should be significant. Think of someone you trust and ask them if they would be willing to talk with you to help you process the issue.

Choose a setting for the conversation that ensures privacy and prevents interruptions. Remember this kind of vulnerability can feel like stepping outside your comfort zone, and be kind to yourself for taking this step.

prompt ■ ■

When we want to make another person feel special, we consider what brings them pleasure. What are some things you can do to care for yourself and add a little joy to your life?

Write a Love Letter

In the business of life, we often forget to tell others how much we appreciate them—we take each other for granted. Making time to pause and think about the ways others enrich our lives can lift our mood. Our circle of support, no matter how large or small, can provide a sense of safety and comfort.

For this practice, you will write a letter (or even an email or text message) expressing your gratitude to anyone in your orbit. It doesn't have to be a friend—you can also write to a coffee shop barista or mailman. You aren't committing to sending the message, and you can always decide to share this letter with them later.

As you write, consider the gifts, gestures, or assistance this person has given you. Which specific acts have touched you? Be as generous as possible! After you're done, make note here of how you feel.

Check-In

At this point, do you have a new or different appreciation for how your relationships affect your quality of life? Which mindfulness practices have had a positive effect on your social well-being?

Playful Creativity

As busy adults, playing or being creative may be low on our list of priorities. This is unfortunate, as play and creativity can bring us into the present while providing relief from life's stresses—and can even be used as tools for problem-solving. Here, we'll welcome more playfulness and creativity into our lives.

Find some colorful writing tools and blank paper. (If you didn't have such supplies as a child, allow yourself to enjoy what's available now—look at the range of colors available for play!)

Notice which colors you like most and be sure to use them in your creation. Start "coloring." You can doodle or draw; it doesn't matter. Notice any thoughts and feelings that arise and let them pass by. How does playful creativity feel in your body? Do you find yourself judging yourself or this exercise? Can you feel a sense of freedom or fun?

Think of your childhood and all your favorite activities. Where did you like to spend time? What were your favorite toys? Whom did you play with? How can these memories inspire you to be creative and find time for play now?

RAIN

RAIN is a powerful practice for when you feel stuck on thoughts or flooded with intense emotions. It provides a way to acknowledge and release the energy of our emotions and ends with self-care, increasing our capacity to manage our feelings and fully engage with life. Allow at least 15 minutes for this practice.

R   Recognize an emotion. Notice any additional feelings that surface.

A   Allow the feeling(s) to be. Imagine making space for whatever arises—no need to resist, judge, or act.

I   Investigate what's happening. Bring curiosity (see page 84) to the moment. What thoughts or urges first came to mind? What did you want to do? As you let those urges go, what did you notice next?

N   Nurture yourself with compassion. Be "nice" to yourself—opening yourself to exploring challenging moments is hard and requires loving care. Ask yourself what you can do to be kind to yourself.

Now that you understand how mindfulness practices help us recognize, accept, and work with thoughts and feelings, what steps can you take NOW to support mindfulness in your life?

Being mindful
allows me to be more
present, manage
my emotions
with compassion, and
experience more
peace and pleasure
in life.

Resources

Websites

Dr. Kristin Neff's Self-Compassion website shares compassion exercises as well as guided meditations. Her Self-Compassion Break is Exercise 2 on the website. **Self-Compassion.org/category/exercises**.

Mental Health America releases an annual report tracking trends within the United States. It also evaluates mental health services available within each state. **MHANational.org/issues/state -mental-health-america**.

The Mindfulness-Based Stress Reduction (MBSR) Training website explains MBSR and provides access to a range of mindfulness exercises. **MBSRTraining.com**.

Dr. Steven C. Hayes, the founder of Acceptance and Commitment Therapy (ACT), offers a free ACT toolkit. **StevenCHayes.com**.

The Values in Action Institute on Character offers a free, online self-assessment tool that provides a report of your character strengths. **VIACharacter.org**.

Apps for iOS and Android Devices

InsightTimer.com. Insight Timer has over 80,000 free recordings, including guided meditations, talks, multi-day courses, music tracks, and links to podcast interviews.

UCLAHealth.org/marc/ucla-mindful-app. The University of California at Los Angeles (UCLA) Mindful Awareness Research Center's UCLA Mindful app offers meditations, instructional videos, and podcasts.

References

Brach, Tara. *Radical Compassion: Learning to Love Yourself and Your World with the Practice of RAIN.* London: Penguin Life, 2020.

Canady, Valerie A. "MHA Annual State Report Finds Rising MH Rates Pre-COVID." *Mental Health Weekly* 30, no. 41 (2020). doi.org/10.1002/mhw.32558.

Hamilton, David R. *Why Kindness Is Good for You.* Carlsbad, CA: Hay House, 2010.

Hill, Diana, and Debbie Sorensen. *ACT Daily Journal: Get Unstuck and Live Fully with Acceptance and Commitment Therapy.* Oakland: New Harbinger Publications, 2021.

Kraft, Tara L., and Sarah D. Pressman. "Grin and Bear It: The Influence of Manipulated Facial Expression on the Stress Response." *Psychological Science* 23, no. 11 (2012): 1372–78. doi.org/10.1177/0956797612445312.

Linehan, Marsha M. *DBT Skills Training Handouts and Worksheets.* New York: Guilford Press, 2014.

Neff, Kristin, and Christopher Germer. *The Mindful Self-Compassion Workbook: A Proven Way to Accept Yourself, Build Inner Strength, and Thrive.* New York: Guilford Press, 2018.

———. "The Transformative Effects of Mindful Self-Compassion." *Mindful.* January 29, 2019. Mindful.org/the-transformative-effects-of-mindful-self-compassion.

Peck, M. Scott. *The Road Less Traveled: A New Psychology of Love, Traditional Values, and Spiritual Growth*. New York: Simon and Schuster, 2002.

Yang, Larry. *Awakening Together: The Spiritual Practice of Inclusivity and Community*. Somerville, MA: Wisdom Publications, 2017.

Acknowledgments

This is for my mother, my family, and my children for loving me despite my imperfections. I'm thankful to my clients for allowing me into their lives. My work is shaped by my teachers, Jack Kornfield and Tara Brach, and the mentorship of Rebecca Hines. Most importantly, I am where I am because of the support of my husband, Ron, who shares my appreciation of mindfulness.

About the Author

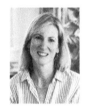

Elizabeth Cronin, PsyD, is a clinical psychologist and certified mindfulness meditation teacher in private practice in Brookline, Massachusetts. She is a podcast host for The New Books Network psychology and mindfulness channels. She has a doctorate degree from William James College and a master's degree from the Harvard University Graduate School of Education. For more information, visit drelizabethcronin.com.